NCLEX EXAM

What You Need To Know Before You Take Your Exam

By

Chioma Okeke

Table of Contents

About the book

This book was created for individuals testing to take the National Council

Licensure Examination. The contents within this book are original with need to

know information to prepare for the exam in addition to understanding what to

expect.

Copyright

Author

Chioma Okeke

Preface

The exit point into nursing has been established by an exam known as the National Council Licensure Examination (NCLEX). The format of the distribution of this exam has evolved with up and coming changes in technology, however the principle of the exam has not changed. This book was created as a how to manual of key specifics nurses need to know prior to taking their exam as well as ways in which they can prepare.

About the Author

Chioma Okeke is a licensed Registered Nurse with a Bachelor's of Science Degree in Nursing. She is also an established writer and the founder of Choosing Nursing at choosingnursing.net where she provides additional advice and resources for nurses and nursing students. She prides herself in helping new nurses successfully transition into the nursing field. She is also a contributor for NurseTogether.com.

What Is The NCLEX?

The National Council Licensure Exam (NCLEX) is a computer adaptive test that nurses who have graduated from an accredited nursing school must successfully pass in order to be licensed to work as a registered nurse or a licensed practical nurse. Originally the exam was a paper test exam dated back to 1994 and at that time nurses had to wait weeks before obtaining their results. Imagine not knowing if you passed or failed your NCLEX exam until weeks later.

Now with advances in the new technology age, nurses can receive their results within the same day (Pearson Vue trick) to a few days. The purpose of the exam is for nurses to demonstrate if they are a safe and competent nurse to practice in the field. Changes to the exam are made approximately every three years (sometimes more frequently), with the most recent change in 2015 where Canada now also recognizes the NCLEX as their license exit exam which was previously the Canadian Registered Nurse Examination (CRNE).

The National Council of State of Boards in Nursing (NCSBN) composes the exam by interviewing thousands and thousands of registered nurses to create the content on the exam.

There are two types of NCLEX examinations. There is the NCLEX-RN exam and there is the NCLEX-PN exam. The NCLEX-RN exam is specifically for nurses who want to obtain a license as a registered nurse. Due to the increase in the level of education required to become a registered nurse, the NCLEX-RN exam is subsequently known to be more difficult than the NCLEX-PN exam. The NCLEX-RN exam is also based on the increase in the scope of practice that registered nurses can do as opposed to licensed practical nurses. The NCLEX-PN exam is for nurses who desire to obtain a license as a licensed practical nurse or LPN.

Testing Time

The NCLEX-RN exam has a tested time frame of 6 hours maximum in time. The NCLEX-PN exam has a time frame of 5 hours maximum in time. The number of questions one can be tested on the exam is a minimum of 75 questions to a maximum of 265 questions. The number of questions obtained on the exam is not a direct indicator of whether one has passed or failed the exam. The exam is adaptive towards the test takers responses to the questions so not every individual's exam is the same. In addition the number of questions you obtain on the exam is not the same.

The Contents On The Exam

The specific contents seen on the NCLEX exam is listed for your convenience below. Physiological integrity comprises a large percentage on the exam.

1. Physiological Integrity

- Basic Care and Comfort

- Pharmacological and Parenteral Therapies

- Reduction of Risk Potential

2. Physiological Adaptation

3. Safe Effective Care Environment

4. Management of Care

5. Safety and Infection Control

6. Health Promotion and Maintenance

7. Psychosocial Integrity

International Nurses

An individual with a degree in nursing, can test for the National Council Licensure Exam within the United States even if they did not attain their degree within the United States. They must however look up the specific requirements to obtain their license in the state they wish to be licensed in prior to attempting to schedule for their NCLEX exam. Unfortunately statistically speaking, nurses who test for the NCLEX exam that have obtained their degree outside of the United States are known to have a lower passing rate, *even* if they have experience working as a nurse in their country. There are multitude of reasons why this could be.

For one the level of difficulty of the exam may be greater than the type of curriculum they are accustomed to. Another reason this may be is because the healthcare system within their country may not be the same as the healthcare system of the United States. Due to this it is very important that nurses who obtained their degree outside of the U.S. and wish to obtain there license should be more rigorous in preparing for their NCLEX exam.

Where To Find Secrets About The Exam

Oftentimes when nurses are preparing for the NCLEX exam, they become so overwhelmed with all the content they need to know but they learn very little about the actual exam. Information that could easily help guide them and equip them with valuable insights to better help them prepare.

One of the best ways to learn more about the National Licensure Council Exam is to go to the ones who created it. The ones who designed the exam which is the National Council State of Boards in Nursing (NCSBN). The NCSBN lists significant information about the NCLEX exam on the website (https://ncsbn.org/). Aside from only reviewing what to expect the day of your exam, you can also learn other specifics or "secrets" about the questions as well as the material on the exam. Here are three specifics about the exam that you may or may not already be aware of.

1. For all the calculation questions (such as drug dosage calculations) always round the calculation at the very end of the calculation not at the beginning or throughout your calculation.

2. For pharmacology (medications) the exam will mainly test on the generic name of the drug more often than the brand name. Example: Furosemide is the generic name vs Lasix which is the brand or trade name.

3. Multiple response items questions, also known as select all questions, requires at least two or more answers in order for the answer to be correct. Therefore do not choose one answer only. This is helpful in identifying the answers for these questions.

These are just a few of the facts on the exam that is very helpful to know prior to studying for this test. I encourage you to go through their website and explore it for other more valuable information when you are testing for the exam.

How To Prepare For It

Okay so now it's that time. Time to take your NCLEX exam. But how do you prepare for it? How do you tackle this exam and study it so you can pass? What is and how is the BEST way to prepare for the NCLEX exam? Well I am going to get right into how to study for the NCLEX.

First I do want to address some things because what I'm going to suggest is not necessarily going to apply to everyone, *ideally*. Here are two main examples where these suggestions may not work as well and what you can do about it.

The Exceptions

First as mentioned before, is if you received your nursing education outside of the United States. Unfortunately as mentioned in chapter one "What Is The NCLEX?", nurses who obtain their degree outside of the U.S have a significantly much lower passing rate. As of 2015, the NCLEX pass rate for first time international nurse test takers is only **31.49%!** I know this is such an alarming rate. If you are an international student and you're reading this, I don't want you to lose hope. But you do need to realize that you will need more preparation, more studying than your local counterparts.

Some international nurses may also struggle with English comprehension. Even those who have lived in the United States all their lives still struggle with what the exam is actually asking them so there may be a gap in the level of English proficiency required for international nurses to understand the exam.

For some states within the United States (not all) they actually require for international nurses to sit through another exam (a certification) before they can they even *take* the NCLEX-RN exam. You need to look into the state of boards nursing you would like to be licensed in and see if they have this requirement. One of the requirements some of these states may require for international nurses is a type of certification. This is called the CGFNS Certification Program. This certification is a qualifying exam of demonstration of English language proficiency for international nurses. You can learn more information about this program and their services through their website www.cgfns.org.

The other unique situation is if it's been years since you've graduated nursing school but have been unable to pass, once again you will also need a higher level of preparation to successfully pass the exam the next time. Depending on the type of education you received you may benefit from completing a RN Refresher course first to refresh your memory of nursing, update you with new practices as well as promote new critical thinking.

If however you did fail the exam within the past year or if you want more specific insights on *why* nurses do not pass their exam , then I do have a free guide to help you. You can access it by going to http://choosingnursing.net. It is called "10 NCLEX Mistakes You Must Avoid So You Don't Fail Your Exam". This is a great resource for you to get started with.

What I Did

Now I'm going to tell you exactly what I did to pass and pass the first time. This may or may not work for you but overall I believe this is effective. I also HIGHLY recommend studying in study groups.

- Set a NCLEX test date up to three months from the time of your graduation. The longer you wait, the lower your chances are of passing. This is very important.

- Study with a few resources and manage your time well. I recommend using one Saunder's book of practice questions, one review course , your medical surgical book (the big one) and or a Kaplan review book (In the next chapter I discuss which books specifically).

- Devote time to study and time to relax (you don't want to burn yourself out). Obviously the time you spend studying should be greater than the total time you're relaxing.

- I didn't waste my time reading forums and online nurse stories. Honestly to me it only takes away from your time when you could be using it studying and focusing. There may be some resources on there but it's not very effective spending much of your time on there.

- BEGIN your studying by taking a practice exam to identify right now if you were to take the exam TODAY how you would do. This is crucial because it will allow you to identify where you are most weak in. Once you identify these areas go back to your medical surgical book and STUDY those areas.

Contrary to what you may think, taking only NCLEX practice questions every day until you take the exam is not the best way to prepare (In the upcoming chapter "What To DO With Practice Questions" I discuss this more in detail). You need to see how you are really doing at the beginning, the middle, the middle again and towards the end. There's this powerful quote that goes "What gets measured, gets managed" by William Thomson. This is true. You need to measure how you're doing to see if you are doing well. Otherwise, all you're really doing is going into the NCLEX underprepared. This is what I did, I took a practice test at the beginning of my studying (did poorly) then again right before I took the exam (huge improvement difference). The NCLEX exam *is* hard, it is challenging, but it is also doable. And you can pass it with the right preparation.

Top 3 NCLEX Review Books

If you are currently in a position right now where you are preparing to study for your NCLEX exam and you're ready and willing to invest in some resources to help you pass then that is what we will be discussing now. In this chapter, I highlight my top three NCLEX review books that I have personally used and recommend. I outline the reasons why I recommend them so you can have some kind of direction on which books may be right for you.

Saunders (A Must Have)

Saunders Q & A Review for the NCLEX-RN® Examination, 4e (Silvestri, Saunders Q & A Review for the NCLEX-RN Examination) 4th Edition by Linda Anne Silvestri PhD RN (Author) on Amazon for $5.37.

It is highly recommended that you invest in at least one Saunders Review book. Saunders review books are excellent at providing you with questions that mirror the questions on the NCLEX exam. In addition, they provide detailed rationales to each of the questions so it explains the answers to each question. This not only exposes you to more NCLEX like questions but it also invokes critical thinking so that way you know how to answer each question, every single time. I specifically enjoyed this book because it helped me to identify if I was really ready for the NCLEX exam by taking notice of how many questions I was missing.

Pros: Ideal to judge how well you understand the questions enough to pass the NCLEX exam.

Also very helpful in preparing you for the difficulty level of the NCLEX exam questions.

Cons: It is a question based book so if you want to have a better understanding of the material topics itself you need to use another resource.

Prentice Hall Nursing

Prentice-Hall Nursing Reviews & Rationales: Medical-Surgical Nursing, 2nd Edition 2nd Edition by Mary Ann Hogan (Author), Stacy Estridge (Author), Dolores Zygmont (Author), Joan Davenport (Author) on Amazon for $17.85

This book is by far AMAZING if you are weak in your understanding of Medical Surgical Nursing (which by the way is a large component of the exam). This book is a great place to start if you recently graduated nursing school and you need more insight in the medical surgical area. I loved this book because it literally connected the dots of things I was missing and not grasping. It condenses everything you need to know about Medical Surgical nursing and provides you with the critical thinking that helps you to successfully pass the NCLEX exam. Highly recommended.

Pros: Ideal to build your foundation in the medical surgical area so you can critically think through the exam.

Cons: Limited number of NCLEX practice questions

Kaplan Review

NCLEX-RN Content Review Guide by Kaplan on Amazon for $37.78

Now this book is more pricier than the other books but I promise you that it's worth it. This book is from Kaplan. First let me say one advantage with the Kaplan books is that they not only have one for NCLEX-RN but they also have one for NCLEX-PN.

The Kaplan books are very excellent because it's more comprehensive than most review books. It provides the actual content for you to study and to better learn from. So for example in one section you can learn what you need to know about maternity nursing (content) and in addition the book comes with a very helpful CD. You can also utilize their website for a limited number of practice questions. Still highly recommend even if you decide not to take their preparation review course.

Pros: Very comprehensive guide of nearly everything you need to know to study the exam.

Cons: Limited number of NCLEX practice questions.

*If you noticed, these are all old editions for when I myself was taking the exam, so I highly recommend that if you can, to obtain these books in their *newest* edition today but if you cannot the older editions are still an excellent resource. The images of all these books are listed on http://choosingnursing.net

5 Free NCLEX Tools To Help You Study

One of the biggest problems a lot of nursing students have is their ability to understand all of the content and the material necessary to pass the NCLEX exam. There is SO MUCH information and content to cover so understanding the material can be very overwhelming. Here are **_5 FREE TOOLS_** that will not only help you study throughout nursing school but will also help you pass your NCLEX exam.

The first tool is an application or app. The purpose of this app is to be an online flashcard tool. For those of you who like to save paper, or don't want to buy index cards you are going to love this tool. This app is called Chegg Flashcards. It is available for download on iOS. It may or may not be available for download on a Android phone. The beauty of this app is you can literally categorize your flashcards into different topics as well as create individual online flash cards that you can study from.

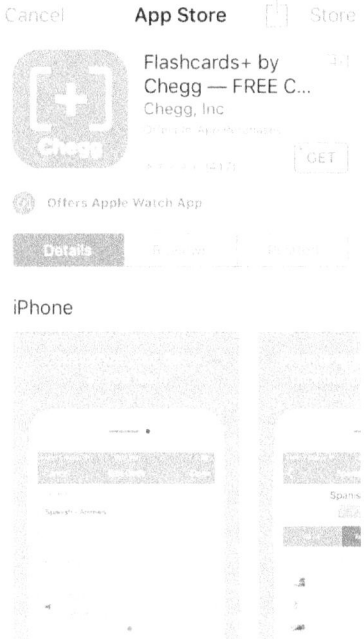

The previous picture is what the app looks like. Once you download the app for free, the next image is what you will see. Except the word pharmacology won't be there, because it is added in for demonstration. You would then choose "Create deck" so you can create one large category of the type of flash cards you want to be in this deck. The example given for you below is pharmacology.

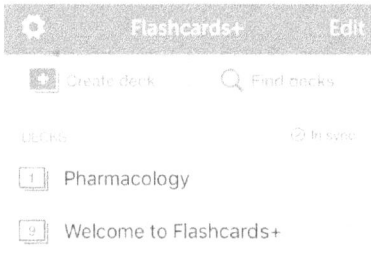

After you have created your deck, then you can begin to create individual flash cards inside. This is what the screen will then look like.

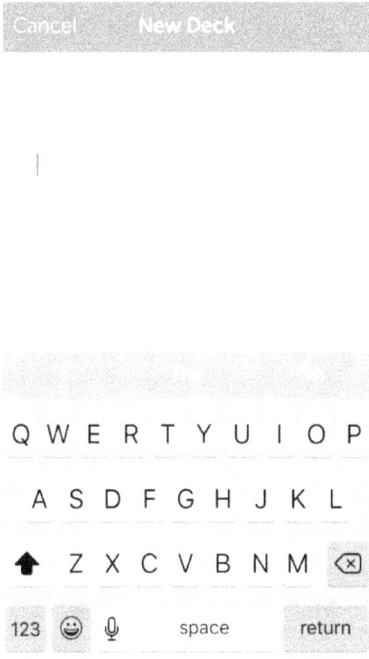

The other wonderful thing about this app is that it's very handy for images that you want to insert in as well as other visual aids to help you remember the picture. In addition you can also use it to screenshot from other online resources, such as a study guide, and insert it, in order to better help you retain the material.

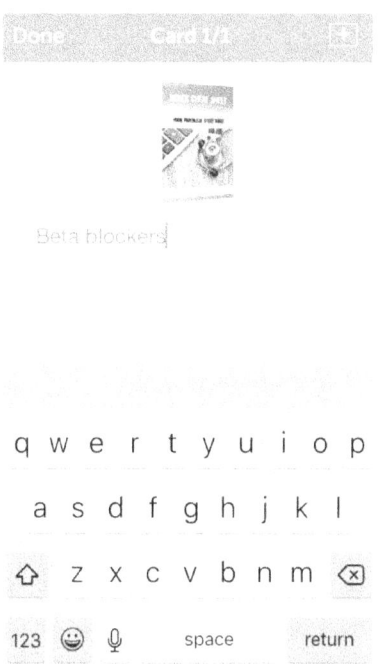

In the image above, the top is a picture of the NCLEX Cheat Sheet Study Guide for the front of card and the back says "beta blockers". Another example could be the front of the card says "Furosemide" and the back of the card could say "diuretics that decreases the potassium level".

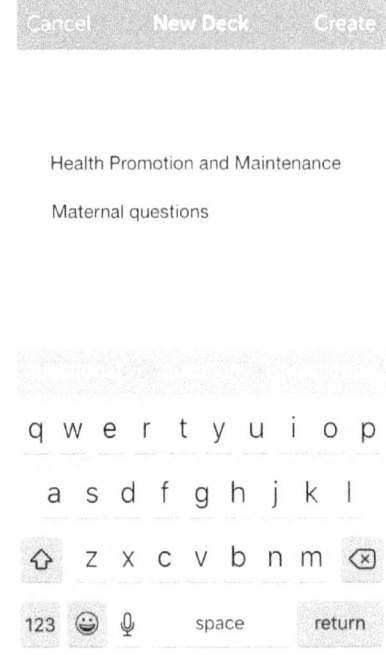

Another example is the front of the card says "Health Promotion and Maintenance and the back of the card says "Maternal Questions" as seen in the image above. This app is a great way to use flash cards on your phone without having to actually spend hours writing out flashcards as well as buying index cards. I encourage you to use it when you are studying for your NCLEX exam.

Acadoodle

The next tool is called acadoodle at acadoodle.com. Now not all of the resources on this website is free but it may be worth the cost given the value of the free information they give you. If you are a visual learner as well as if you need the material broken down in a way for you to better retain the material, then you are going to love this website. It includes topics such as EKGs, Arterial Blood Gases, and more. They have video courses that you can pay for if you sign up however it does have a great amount of free videos as well.

Picmonic

The next free tool is called Picmonic at picmonic.com. Now Picmonic is completely visual and video. It makes the material plain by using interactive videos, cartoon like images and easy to understand language for the content. With Picmonic you can choose to see the categories in nursing you want to master or understand better. For example you can choose to learn more about the nursing process as seen as above. When you choose a topic such as the nursing process, you have the option to either listen which means that you listen to what the content is telling you, then you can go into learning mode which is where you are reviewing the material and contents you just listened/watched. Then finally is Master mode where you literally test yourself through the interactive video to see if you have actually mastered the content. Picmonic is extremely visual and I believe they also have an app as well. However I recommend using them via your desktop in order to get the full access to the resources. This is another great free tool to help you understand the content in a more layman's term.

Evernote

The next free tool is called Evernote at evernote.com. Now Evernote is by no means a resource that's going to teach you how to study nursing, the material on the NCLEX exam, or anything like that. However it is extremely ideal in order for you to be organized with your study notes, presentation, and any other valuable information you need to collect as you are studying. Evernote keeps you organized so that way you're not all over the place with the things you need to study. For example you can utilize this tool to group your presentations that you are learning or have learned in your classes. You can group all the notes you have taken from a specific subject area. You can also group everything you need to do to study for your exam.

For example:

"I need to buy more pencils and pens".

"I need to schedule my exam".

"I need to apply for my ATT".

Notes such as this is the ideal purpose of Evernote which is to help really keep you organized.

Jones & Bartlett's Nurse's Drug Handbook App

The next and final tool is called *Jones & Bartlett Nurse Drug Handbook* and this is once again found on your iOS phone. This app may also be on a Android device too. The app is just straight clinical pharmacology only. So if pharmacology is something you are really really struggling with and you do not understand it at all, this app may be beneficial for you. This app is a drug handbook app for nurses. So it really has ALL of the medications you could possibly need to know as a nurse. It's very convenient and you can look up everything you need to know for specific drugs.

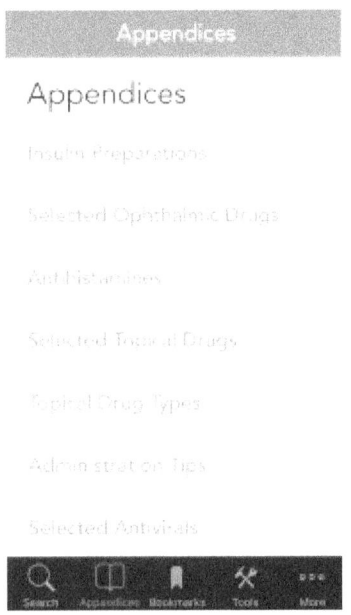

As you can see from the picture, the medications are categorized to specific groups so that way you can pick categories to review the drugs and gain a better understanding. This is also a great app to use when you begin working as a nurse which means you can utilize it for not just only when you are studying for the NCLEX exam. Since you can pull out your phone (if your facility permits it) you can quickly find a specific drug with all of the necessary indications you need to know about that drug. This is a great free tool if you are looking to strengthen your understanding of pharmacology.

What To Do With Practice Questions

Many people have different ways of tackling NCLEX practice questions but what people struggle with is the HOW. You can by all means do 100 questions a day everyday until you take your exam and that may work for you but I'm going to tell you right now that's not the purpose of NCLEX practice questions.

The purpose of NCLEX practice questions is to identify your level of comprehension of the material *through* the questions not just your ability to answer as many questions as correctly as possible. If you're doing questions just to do questions and you're not identifying with the rationales then there's a gap in your studying. Practice questions are excellent because they should teach you *how* to answer NCLEX questions (if they're true NCLEX like questions). If you're doing multiple types of practice questions and you're scoring low then that simply means you don't understand the material. However you still need to do NCLEX questions that really mirror the questions on the NCLEX exam otherwise you're going to be blind-sighted when you take the exam.

Types of NCLEX Practice Questions

A great way to breakdown NCLEX practice questions is into two different categories. There are NCLEX practice questions that you do out of a book (ex: Saunders book). Then there's NCLEX practice questions you do on a computer (in test mode). You need to do both especially practice questions on a computer. If you're just doing it out of a book, you're not really preparing yourself very well for the exam because without it, it's not teaching you *how* the NCLEX exam tests you.

For example doing it on a computer, familiarizes you with taking NCLEX questions on a computer screen. It familiarizes you with doing questions one after the other in test mode rather than flipping between the rationale answers with the questions in a book.

My Recommendation

One of things I like to do is I spend time searching for NCLEX practice questions to help nurses I work with. I have recently done a lot of practice questions myself just so I can find the best ones out there. I have used several different sources of NCLEX practice questions that's available. Almost all of them are good, but I haven't been able to find questions that really mirrors the same questions on the NCLEX exam. Until now...

BrilliantNurse is by far in my opinion one of the BEST websites that houses and mirrors the questions on the NCLEX Exam. I took many of their practice exam questions and by far I was impressed. As I started researching them more, I found out that they are actually a company owned by nurses! Of course! Now it makes sense who else better to illustrate NCLEX like questions than fellow nurses themselves.

If you would like to give them a try you can begin by taking some of their free NCLEX questions. They also offer a large number of questions for a great value. For example they have a pool of NCLEX questions for only $35 for 3500 questions. I know that many people are spending much more for NCLEX practice questions but with less number of questions so I was very glad when I found them as a resource.

What Happens When You Pass

Congratulations! You passed. Or maybe you're just wondering what exactly happens when you pass your NCLEX exam. You will know if you passed your exam by simply going to the Board of Registered Nursing for the state you applied to (the web address is specific to your state). On the website, you will be able to enter in your full name where you should see "PASS" next to your name as well as your newly licensed number. Write this number down but you will receive it weeks later on your license card in the mail. You can notify your employer that you passed your exam and they can look up your name and license through the website. Once you receive your license in the mail, it's very important that you keep it safe inside your wallet at all times.

License Renewal

You will need to renew your license every two years thus after by obtaining at least 30 continuing education units(CEUs). This is not difficult at all because there will be multiple opportunities where you will be able to obtain CEUs especially through your employer.

But now you can relax. You never have to worry about taking the exam again. You did it!

The Number One Mistake Why Nurses Fail Their NCLEX Exam

I know how frustrating and challenging it is to prepare for something you've never done before. Even no matter how many similar practice exams you may take; it still doesn't change the fact that it's not going to be the exact same test on your test date.

I know for me personally I had so much anxiety preparing for this exam. And it wasn't just me; I had a family waiting for me to PASS. I had student loan bills I knew I was going to have to pay soon and a desire to finally be independent and be on my own making my own money. I was so scared. And I can only imagine how disheartening it must be to take this particular test and be forced to take it again and again. Like most people, there are other individuals besides yourself who are waiting and hoping for you to pass. Whether it may be your spouse so that there will be two incomes coming into the household or maybe you have children to take care of, it's the growing norm of life. We all have people who are connected to us that are dependent upon our success.

Take for example Jennifer.

Jennifer just finished nursing school with her bachelor's degree. She is married to her husband who currently works as a security guard. Jennifer is very excited to soon start working in hopes that her and her husband can soon purchase a new house. She is currently working a CNA job to help pay the bills and has a $62,380 loan debt from her bachelor's degree in nursing.

Prior to taking the exam, Jennifer was studying in study groups with her fellow classmates who have now already passed the exam. She bought two nurse review books and has been using flash cards from resources she found from online quizzes. After six weeks of studying, Jennifer decides she's ready to take her NCLEX exam. Feeling confident, she finishes the exam after 195 questions. Within a short few days, Jennifer is heartbroken to discover she FAILED her exam. Not only does she feel like she let down herself, but also her family as well.

While browsing online, Jennifer stumbles upon the 10 NCLEX Mistakes You Must Avoid So You Don't Fail Your Exam. She identifies with Mistake #6 (**in report**) and the #1 Mistake. She becomes inspired again and decides to take the exam ONE more time. Previously skeptical before due to the cost, she enrolls in a review course. It is through the course she is able to identify her weak areas preventing her from passing the NCLEX. She finishes the course. Three days after her test date, she checks the Board of Registered Nursing website and sees her name next to the word "RN"….Jennifer is elated! Within a short amount of time, she lands herself a position at a prestigious hospital where both her and her husband now reside in a nearby suburban neighborhood.

So you want to know what I found is the Number #1 **BIGGEST** reason why nurses do not pass the NCLEX exam?

No prep course.

Now this is not to say that there aren't nurses who are passing *without* taking a prep course but this might be the reason why some are not. I HIGHLY recommend taking a prep course if you haven't done so or if you keep failing or both. And sometimes the problem isn't always that nurses are not taking a prep course at all, but that they're not completing it in its *entirety.* They're electing to take the smallest version of the review course or they're starting it but not finishing. You

HAVE to complete it from beginning to the end. A small investment is going to always get you a small return.

And just like not taking a prep course, there are other common completely oblivious mistakes nurses are making that are setting themselves up for **FAILURE** when preparing for their NCLEX exam. The trick is to learn those mistakes **BEFORE** you start preparing. And if you're thinking, I'm only in my second semester of nursing school, I don't need to know this.

WRONG. This is information you want to be aware of at *any* stage in nursing school. Because guess what, your program may be hard, but I can assure you it's going to go by **FAST.** So why not prep yourself now? In the 10 NCLEX Mistakes To Avoid So You Don't Fail Your Exam I line out what those key mistakes are that you may be making or *could* make. Mistakes that may be blocking your chances of SUCCESS. You can click on the link above to have your report within seconds.

Now……. let me tell you about one prep course I took in the past (Kaplan). One of the biggest things I enjoyed about this review is that it begins by identifying your weak areas first by instructing you to take an initial diagnostic test. This allows you to *hone* in on your weak points and strengthen your strong points. Once it identifies your weaknesses, it provides strategic material to strengthen those weaknesses. Then when you feel ready, after a series of studying the structured material they provide; you can take their diagnostic test again and again and again, so that you can literally see and track your progress.

Doing practice review questions over and over again is great but it doesn't allow you to see where you're lacking in your studying ESPECIALLY if you've been failing. If you've been failing and you've been failing more than once, it's not always necessarily the case that you don't know nursing but rather that you don't know how to *apply* it so that the exam believes you're a competent nurse.

But you have to know right now and believe right now that **THIS** could be a game changer for you. There's still hope. No matter if this is your first or your fifth time, you CAN pass this exam.

I did it and now so can YOU.

It's knowing that there are root causes as to why nurses fail their NCLEX exam, so it's not you, it's something that you're doing (or not doing). And once you know what these reasons are then you can begin to take the right measures to overcome them.

What To Do If You Failed The NCLEX Exam

As of last year the NCSBN reported there were approximately 12 to 14% US-based nurses who did not pass the NCLEX-RN exam in the year of 2015. The number 14% may not seem like that many nurses, but also keep in mind there are over hundreds of thousands of nurses who are entering into the nursing field and almost 3 million nurses inside the United States. So 14% can actually be a large number of nurses who did not pass the exam the first time in 2015.

The first thing I want to tell you is that if this is you, you can first breathe, you can relax. I know it seems like the end of the world but I promise you that it's not. There are plenty of nurses who were unsuccessful with passing the exam on the first try or even multiple times, and have went on to have very successful careers in nursing. They still go on to work, they still go on to become charge nurses, preceptors and managers so you don't have to feel as though failing one time or more will hinder you from becoming a great nurse. It's not always a matter of how many times it takes you to get there, just as long as you get there. So I want to encourage you right now that it's not the end of the world, you just have to make some choices where you do things differently in order to make sure that you pass the next time. Because there is a saying that goes that if you keep doing the same thing over and over again you're only going to get the same result. So it's the exact same thing.

What Happens Next

If you did not pass then you will have to wait 45 days before you can retest for the exam again. It is important that you get your results even if you did not pass your exam so that you can see what areas you are struggling with. You can identify what areas you are scoring "above passing", "near passing" and/or "below passing". This is very significant so that you can begin improving in these areas. You may also need to get a new Authorization to Test (ATT). The Authorization to Test is something you receive prior to taking your NCLEX exam to permit your eligibility to take the exam through the Board of Nursing. The average length of time for an ATT is usually 90 days. If yours expires and you still have not passed your exam, you will need to reapply for another one.

Different Measures

The next thing is there are different measures that you need to take if you failed one time as opposed to if you failed two or more times. However everybody is different, not everything discussed is going to be cut and dry for everybody. This is only general advice to follow by. One of the reasons why is because I cannot calculate what type of the strategies you implemented the first time or the amount of effort you did while you were studying. Therefore this is why there is not one blanket answer for everybody. This is just something that I have found for some people.

For some people if you didn't pass the first time you may just need to be more aggressive with your studying the next time and implement more strategies the next time in order to be successful in passing when you take your exam again. Some people just need that extra studying time, that extra time going over the content and the material. They may not have done as much studying as they know they could have done the first time they took their exam.

Now if you have failed two times or more, then this requires a higher level of investment. Because the more times you go without passing the exam, the longer it takes you to pass your exam, then the less likely you are to eventually pass. One of the things that I mean by a higher level of investment may include putting more time for example. You going to need to invest more of your time to help you get the results you want. You may need to sacrifice some things in order to allot this time. Keep in mind that this is only a temporary season it's not forever.

You're also going to have to invest in more resources, not too many resources, but however the right ones. Some people may only need a Saunders book to read through front and back and can pass the exam the next time whereas others may need to invest at a higher level and seek out tutors, review courses, or other outside help for them to get to the end result. It really depends on the person as well as how many times they have taken the exam. Some people really need more hand-holding, they need more personalized attention, they need more insight and strategies in order to help them see the whole picture. Everyone is different.

Get Help

However one thing that I do believe is that the sooner you get help, regardless of how many times you have taken your exam, the more likely you are to pass. So the sooner you get help, the higher your chances are of passing sooner than later. For me personally I remember that I was willing to invest whatever it took. I did not help of a mentor to bridge the gap of the need of nurses struggling to pass or prepare for their exam. If you are currently looking for help to pass your NCLEX exam whether it be the first time or you've exhausted all your other resources then this may be the program for you. One thing I pride myself is that I am very passionate about what I do and LOVE doing this. I've been a Registered Nurse now for six years in the area of Medical Surgical and Telemetry nursing and this is what I have devoted myself to doing. Helping other nurses get exactly to where I am by teaching them how to pass their NCLEX exam. If you need help and this sounds like the program for you then email me and I will do my best to help you.

Thank you so much for reading and don't hesitate to review this book over and over again if needed so to help you prepare for your exam.

Best Regards,

Chioma Okeke RN,BSN,PHN

Where To Find Additional Help

I hope that everything you have learned thus far in this book has been very helpful to you. I understand that every individual is different so for some people reading information through a helpful book may not be enough. I have encountered a number of people who have reached out to me with different stories and different needs. Many people who have not been successful passing their NCLEX exam despite using a number of resources, review programs and etc. And it absolutely saddens me to see people who went through YEARS of nursing school only to still be unable to pass. And whenever I see a need, that is not being fulfilled, I CREATE it.

I could offer you my email address to reach out to me (nursechioma@choosingnursing.net), however I did not believe that would be enough.

However what I did is I designed my own special program called **Solid Steps To NCLEX Success**. This is an individualized coaching program I designed with the care how much I would have to spend or how much time it would require me, because I was so focused on the end result.

I know sometimes people may not want to make the investment in resources. The way you need to look at it is that the longer it takes, the more time you are losing. And your time is something that you're never going to get back. This is time that you could have been working and making thousands of dollars a month. The average starting pay for a new graduate nurse (depending on the area), is roughly $40,000-$50,000 a year which breaks down to over $3,000 a month. So every month you're not producing that income is a month where you're losing that income. Therefore I encourage you to always consider the resources as an investment.

You also need to act quickly, you need to respond right away. I know it's easy to become so discouraged that you decide you want to take a break from studying and preparing, but if you waste too much time your dreams of becoming a nurse may not happen. The purpose is not to pressure you but it's to incite you to take action sooner than later because the longer you go without passing your exam the less likelihood there is that you will eventually pass the exam.

If you go 6 months, 9 months, a year plus, it will be harder to get back into the groove of studying. Therefore it's important to come up with a plan that you can implement so you can pass your exam soon. If you can come up with a 3 month plan, then that would be ideal to help steer you in the right direction so you can pass. Also the other thing about it is that maybe you do pass your exam five years later but then at that point now you have to really learn the language of nursing all over again *because* of the number of years it took you to get your license. So the sooner you react to it and make the necessary changes, the better likelihood you will have to pass the exam the next time.